Prevent Liver Disease

Prevent Liver problem

Read This Book

Olatundun Solomon

olatundunsolomon@gmai
l.com

The liver is an organ in the body that is very important. It functions in the detoxification of the body and also in the digestion of food. The liver needs a lot of care for it to be healthy. There are many ways disease of the liver can be prevented. These are:

(1). Do not eat animal fat.

Eating of animal fat can make fat to build up in the liver. This can cause fatty liver disease.

(2). Do not practice overeating.

Overeating can cause vomiting. Overeating can

make fat build up to occur in the liver. It is therefore, important not to over eat.

(3). Drink clean water.

Drinking clean water hydrates the body. It can make the liver to function well. Drinking clean water can aid the liver to function well. Drinking dirty water can cause disease causing microorganisms to infect the liver. This can cause disease to the liver.

(4). Exercise.

Exercise can cause excess fat in the body to burn. Exercise can burn fat build up in the liver. Exercise can make the liver to function well.

(5). Eat well cooked food.

Eating well cooked food can prevent disease causing microorganisms from entering the body. This can prevent liver infection.

(6). Do not drink alcohol.

Alcohol can make the liver
not to function well.
Alcohol can cause liver
failure to occur.

(7). Eat vegetables.

Vegetables has vitamins
and minerals that can
make the liver to have
immunity against
infections. Eating
vegetables such as lettuce,

spinach, tomatoes and cabbage are very good for the normal function of the liver.

(8). Eat fruits.

Eating fruits such as mango, apple, pineapple and orange is very good for the body. They have vitamins and minerals that can increase the immunity of the liver against infections.

(9). Take drug correct prescription for the treatment of sickness.

Taking overdose can affect the function of the liver negatively.

(10). Do not put too much sugar in food.

Too much sugar in food that is eaten can cause diabetes mellitus. Diabetes mellitus can affect the function of the liver negatively.

(11). Put little salt in food.

Too much salt in food can affect the function of the

liver negatively. It is therefore, important to put little salt in food.

(12). Eat protein.

Protein foods such as Titus fish, egg, beef, chicken and turkey can make the liver to be well developed. Protein food makes growth and development to occur.

(13). Eat carbohydrates.

Carbohydrates such as whole grains, yam, sorghum and potatoes gives energy to the body. This can make the liver to function well.

(14). Sleep well.

Sleeping well refreshes the body. This can make the liver to be healthy.

(15). Do not smoke.

Smoking has poisonous gases. This can cause toxic effect to the blood. This can lead to toxic effect to the liver.

(16). Be far from air pollution.

Air pollution has toxic gases. This can cause poisonous effect to the blood. This can result to poisonous effect to the liver.

(17). Prevent disease causing microorganisms.

Prevent disease causing microorganisms by not drinking dirty water, by not using used syringes from one person to another in the hospital in the treatment of sickness.

(18). Go to the hospital for check up.

Going to the hospital for check up can make

prevention of liver disease
to occur.

(19). Stay in a well
ventilated area.

Staying in a well
ventilated area can make
the body to have enough
oxygen. This can make the
liver to function well.

(20). Practice personal hygiene.

Taking of bath with clean water and soap can prevent skin infection. This can prevent disease causing microorganisms from entering the body from the skin. This can prevent infection of the liver.

(21). Make sure spoon, plate and fork are clean.

Using clean plate, spoon and fork can prevent disease causing microorganisms not to enter the body. Dirty plate, spoon and fork can have disease causing microorganisms in them that can cause infection of

the liver.